AF484428

Essential Oils for Beginners

56 Best Essential Oil Recipes for Your Health and Beauty

Savannah Gibbs

clarifying purposes only and are owned by the owners themselves, not affiliated with this document.

Table of Contents

Introduction

Essential oils are harvested from sweet-smelling plants. Historically, essential oils have been used for medicinal and healing purposes. Today, they are again gaining in popularity, as consumers are discovering their many great benefits.

This book offers a comprehensive guide to not only understanding essential oils but also learning how to use them. By reading this book, you'll learn

- how to purchase and store oils;

- the best techniques to use to enjoy the aromas and powers of these oils;

- the most commonly used essential oils.

The book will also give you 56 valuable essential oil recipes for

- pain relief;

- acne, skin care, and hair care;

- healing colds and flu;

- reducing anxiety and fatigue;

- allergy relief;

and much more!

Including essential oils in your daily life is easy. This book will walk you through the process, teaching you how to use essential oils for your health and beauty needs.

Chapter 1: Introduction of Essential Oils

To understand the benefits of essential oils, you should know their physical properties. Essential oils come from flowers and plants. They are highly concentrated oils that are extracted from these plants and considered to be the essence of these plants. When used in small amounts, these essential oils can have many benefits.

Brief History of Essential Oils

Historically, essential oils have been used for medicinal and healing purposes. While they are increasingly used today for aromatherapy and alternative or supplemental medicine, they have been used by other cultures and societies to treat everything from sunburn to terminal cancer. Use of essential oils can be dated to the twelfth century in early Middle Eastern civilizations. Some researchers suggest that essential oils were used even earlier, pointing to ancient cave drawings that have been discovered in Europe, suggesting that they were used before Roman times.

Historians agree that ancient Egyptians used and produced essential oils. They believed that smell was the most important sense and could tell you things that your eyes, ears, fingers, and mouth could not. In modern times, recent research has been conducted to learn exactly what can be gained from these oils. Results have been interesting to health practitioners and others who are interested in aromatherapy and medicine. For example, studies have shown that frankincense oil can have a dramatic impact on the body's immune system. Essential oils may help prevent disease and cure illnesses that once seemed incurable. The field of essential oils continues to expand, and new discoveries are being made all the time.

Essential Oil Production

The process of producing essential oils is quite intricate and involves extraction from plants. Two major methods are used: distillation and expression.

The most common essential oils used today are distilled. The entire plant, including the roots, leaves, stems, flowers, seeds, and peels, are put into a distillation machine. The apparatus containing the plant is placed over water, and the steam from that water breaks through the plant material, extracting the oil. Most oils are lighter than water, so they rise to the top of any water during the distillation process.

The expression process is also referred to as cold pressing. Think about how olive oil is made — by extracting oil from the fruit with a cold press. This method works best with essential citrus oils, such as orange, lemon, and bergamot. The rind of the citrus fruit is soaked in warm water, making it easier to express the oil from the plant. When you purchase essential oils, you should know how they were produced. Some people believe that distilled citrus oils will evaporate too quickly, so the expression method should be used for these oils.

Benefits of Essential Oils

Essential oils can be used for many different purposes. If you're interested in establishing a calm mood conducive to work, meditation, relaxation, or even high energy, you can use essential oils for aromatherapy. They are included in a number of bath products, such as soap, candles, and sachets. Whether you're looking for a lavender scent, jasmine, or pine and evergreen at holiday time, you can find essential oils that will fill your home with the fragrances you want.

Besides providing pleasant aromas, essential oils can also be used to help you feel better. For topical applications, you can use such essential oils as menthol and anise to help respiratory function. People have found these oils to be effective in soothing colds and illnesses that interfere with proper breathing. Lavender oil has been used as a natural insect repellent, and rose oil has been used for a mental boost.

There are conflicting reports about the scientific benefits of essential oils. Some medical professionals do not believe they provide any real health benefits, but a great many people have reported feeling better while using them.

You do need to be particularly careful if you have any allergies, as mixing essential oils with medications may be dangerous.

Difference between Fragrance Oils & Essential Oils

You need to understand the difference between essential oils and fragrance oils. Essential oils are completely natural, as they are derived from natural plants, but fragrance oils actually have synthetic chemicals, which makes them artificial. Fragrance oils are usually cheaper, and they do smell good, but you will not get the same health and beauty benefits as you would from essential oils. Always make sure that your essential oils are completely pure.

Chapter 2: How to Use Essential Oils

Those who are intrigued by the beauty and benefits of essential oils might be a bit unsure about how to use them. You can enjoy the aromas and powers of these compounds in many different ways. Knowing how to use essential oils properly will maximize what they can do for you.

Essential Oils in the Bath

One of the best ways to enjoy the aromatic benefits of oils as well as their soothing properties is to add them to a bath. While you're running the bathwater, add a few drops of your favorite essential oil to a dispersing agent, which will help the oil spread through the water. Most people use olive oil, honey, or milk for this purpose. Add the combination to your bath and relax. Besides soothing your stress and anxiety, essential oils in the bath will tone your skin, help relieve muscle soreness, improve circulation, and help your body to detox.

Essential Oils by a Diffuser

Diffusers use ultrasonic waves, cool air, or water vapor to distribute essential oils into the air. Various models of essential oil diffusers are available, but citrus essential oils should not be used in a diffuser.

Essential Oils in a Steam

If you have a cold or a respiratory illness, take advantage of the decongestant and sinus benefits found in essential oils. The best oils to use for this purpose are eucalyptus, lemon, thyme, tea tree, and even peppermint. Boil some water, and put five drops of your favorite essential oil into the pot. Cover your head with a towel and lean over the water, inhaling the steam. Be sure to close your eyes, and don't do this while the water is actively boiling.

Essential Oils for Massage

Essential oils can also be used for a massage, but be sure they are blended into a carrier oil so that they don't cause a reaction on your skin.

Ingestion

Most essential oils are not suitable for ingestion, so use caution. It is a good idea to consult an aromatherapist before consuming any essential oil. Lemon, grapefruit, and peppermint essential oils are generally considered safe for ingestion. A drop can be added to a glass of water or tea to make a refreshing drink, but be sure the oils are therapeutic grade and never ingest undiluted essential oils by mouth.

Essential Oil Products

You can find essential oils in a number of different products, such as face creams, body lotions, massage oil, and shampoo. They will help your skin look and feel younger and toned. They can speed up the healing of wounds and scars, and they can also help you achieve an emotional balance that you would not find using products that don't contain these essential oils.

Carrier Oils

When you're learning how to use essential oils, you need to understand the role and purpose of carrier oils, which are oils that are combined with essential oils to dilute them and carry them into the skin, your bathwater, or the air when you're using them for aromatherapy. Carrier oils have different properties and work best with specific essential oils. Always look for labels when you're making your own essential oil lotions, creams, or other products. You'll find a few of the most common carrier oils below.

• **Olive Oil**: This carrier oil is common and inexpensive. You can usually find it in your local grocery store. Just be sure to use "extra virgin" olive oil. This type has more vitamins and minerals than other olive oil.

• **Coconut Oil**: Cold-pressed coconut oil is another great carrier oil because it has lauric acid, which will help promote healthy skin and hair.

• **Corn Oil**: Corn oil is full of minerals as well as vitamins. It's also considered to be an oil of medium weight.

• **Evening Primrose Oil**: This oil is full of antioxidants, and it'll prolong the shelf life of whatever mixture you make.

• **Grapeseed Oil**: This oil is great for a massage, and it doesn't have a strong scent. Due to a high content of linoleic acid, it even dries quickly.

• **Peanut Oil**: Rich in protein, this oil also has many vitamins and is commonly used as an aromatherapy oil.

• **Jojoba Oil**: This is another oil that can extend the shelf life of your product and works well for dry or oily skin.

• **Sweet Almond Oil**: Sweet almond oil is commonly used because it's rapidly absorbed into your skin and is odorless. It also has linoleic acid, helping to improve blood pressure and cholesterol levels. It's even full of protein.

• **Apricot Kernel Oil**: This oil is a great facial oil because it helps to heal and rejuvenate skin cells.

- **Arnica Oil**: You should not use this oil on broken skin, but it's great for both inflammation and bruising.

- **Sunflower Oil**: Rich in vitamin E, sunflower oil is often used for body oils, massages, and homemade lotions.

These are just some of the carrier oils that can be used, but they're some of the most popular ones due to their benefits.

Buying and Storing Essential Oils

The types of oils you buy and where you buy them depends on what you're looking for. When you want essential oil products for aromatherapy, you can buy them from any number of stores and online retailers. If you want to make your own essential oil creations, or if you are treating a specific condition with the oils, you'll want to purchase therapy-grade oils from a reputable retailer. The more intense the oil grade, the more money you'll spend. Before you buy, consider what you'll be using them for.

To store essential oils, you will need to keep them in dark bottles. Use glass or stainless steel; otherwise, the oils will react to the packaging, and you'll end up with something flawed and altered. It's important to keep these oils out of direct sunlight and heat. If you have the opportunity, shop for essential oils in your local area. You will be able to talk to the retailer about how to care for your oils, and you'll see how they're stored. If you don't have a way to buy them in person, take the time to get to know a reputable vendor online, but only work with someone who receives good reviews from satisfied customers.

How to Use Essential Oils: Safety

Essential oils look and smell pretty and come in very small amounts, but these compounds are extremely powerful. Be careful. Most commercial products are safe to use and come with specific warnings and instructions. You have to be very careful when applying them. Inhaling essential oils comes with very low risk, so using them in a diffuser or to freshen up a room is not difficult. When you're using essential oils on your skin or in your bath, dilute them with dispersing agents and carrier oils. Don't use any oils on your skin that have not been diluted. If you notice any irritations, dilute the oil a bit more. People with allergies and sensitive skin should exercise additional caution.

With all essential oils, make sure you avoid contact with your eyes. If you use them on your face or skin, keep them away from your eyes, and don't ingest them without diluting them. Always wash your hands thoroughly afterward.

Some final tips on how to use essential oils safely: remember that they are extremely flammable. Don't burn down your house trying to make it smell nice. Using essential oils during pregnancy is a topic that is currently being debated by consumers, researchers, and healthcare professionals. Use caution and speak to your doctor. You'll also want to keep essential oils out of reach of children.

Chapter 3: Popular Essential Oils

When planning to use essential oils, the biggest question is what essential oils to buy first. You can usually base this decision on each particular recipe you find, but it's best to have some essential oils on hand. Here are some of the most common ones, with a brief explanation of why you should have them on hand.

Bergamot

An essential oil that originates in citrus trees, bergamot has a pleasing scent that can enhance your sense of peace and happiness, and it's a popular oil for room diffusers. Use it as an antiseptic, an antidepressant, and even as a deodorant, but be careful about using it undiluted on the skin, as it can irritate sensitive skin. Blend it into your bath if you're feeling anxious or fearful.

Cinnamon

Cinnamon is an herb that originated in central Asia and was widely used in healing treatments throughout India and Sri Lanka. It's good for more than flavoring your cider and giving your holiday decorations a burst of seasonal scents. It boosts brain function, increases blood circulation, and helps your body fight off infection. Use cinnamon oil to repel mosquitoes as well. Studies have shown that it's effective in killing larvae.

Clove

Clove essential oil is full of antioxidants and has pain-relieving properties. It is also widely used in dental work. Clove oil has antibacterial, antifungal, and antiseptic characteristics. When used in a diffuser, it helps kill airborne microorganisms. When diluted, it can treat cuts, scrapes, and bites.

Eucalyptus

One of the most common essential oils used by nearly everyone is eucalyptus. You might have been using it for years without realizing it. This oil is found in a number of household, health, and beauty products because it's a powerful agent for clearing up a respiratory illness. It can calm a cough, make your scratchy throat feel better, and help eliminate lung congestion. Just keep in mind that this essential oil is extremely potent, so be sure to keep it away from your eyes.

Frankincense

Frankincense essential oil is known to be great for your skin, and it's also considered to have spiritual properties, with many mental and emotional benefits when used properly. It is used in many topical recipes as well as in a diffuser.

Grapefruit

Some of the most common essential oils come from citrus fruits, which are packed with vitamins, minerals, and antioxidants that help you fight disease. The oil is created by cold pressing the rind of the fruit to extract its essence. Grapefruit oil can help you with your weight loss plans. Drop a bit into your tea, or add it to a smoothie. It has also been useful as an antidepressant. Use it in a diffuser or dilute it and spray on your linens.

Geranium

Taken from the leaves of what might be a favorite flower, geranium essential oil is useful due to its citronellol and geraniol. These compounds influence your brain and nervous system, helping you to control your emotions and resist the temptation to become angry or irritable. *This type of oil may have toxic effects when ingested, so use it as an inhalant or an aromatic.*

Lavender

One of the most popular essential oils, lavender has a beautiful effect on your mind, body, and skin. It's used to help you find balance and peace, and it can also take care of bruises, cuts, rashes, and other skin irritations. Its properties will help you cleanse, whether it's something physical, emotional, or spiritual that needs elimination. For help with sleeping, drop a bit of lavender oil on your pillow, or rub it on your wrists. To stop the pain of an insect bite or a burn, put a bit of lavender oil directly on your skin. It can also treat dandruff if you massage it into your scalp.

Lemon

Lemon essential oil is known to repel insects. It's also a natural cleaner, rejuvenating in a bath, and great aromatherapy. Lemon essential oil is even known to help brighten skin, so it makes a great addition to many topical recipes.

Oregano

Oregano essential oils are high in phenol, which means it's highly effective in cleansing receptor spots of the body. It's most commonly used in the Raindrop Technique for healing. In this process, several drops of oregano essential oil are put on the spine and massaged into the back, which is good for muscle tension and pain and also strengthens your immune system. It contains a number of antioxidant properties. Physically, it will open up your respiratory system and help you breathe. Mentally, it can induce feelings of safety and security.

Peppermint

You won't want to be far from your peppermint essential oil when you have a stomach problem. Whether it's indigestion, nausea, or cramping, peppermint can have an immediate and lasting effect on any digestive or gastrointestinal distress. Peppermint essential oil contains a lot of nutrients and minerals, such as vitamin C and potassium. It's one of the oldest essential oils used today, and the relative ease with which oil can be extracted from the peppermint leaves and bark makes it abundant. Add a drop of peppermint oil to your tea or water to help with digestion. Put it into your bathwater to enjoy the aromatherapy and relax your nerves. You can also rub a bit of peppermint oil into your temples to chase away a headache.

Rosemary

A Mediterranean herb that's popular with Italian and Greek cooking, rosemary oil has more to offer than culinary delights. It's excellent for hair care, stimulating follicle growth, and can be used with shampoo. It also has a positive effect on your mood and provides a burst of energy. Try inhaling it when you're studying, trying to focus on a project, or just need an adrenaline jolt.

Sweet Orange

This great essential oil can be used in your bath, a degreaser, as a lotion, or is even a great oil to diffuse to help you stay focused but relaxed.

Tea Tree

Tea tree oil can help treat skin conditions, and it's a powerful antimicrobial. You should never take it by mouth, though, because it can be toxic. Tea tree oil has nearly one hundred compounds, making it one of the most common and effective essential oils. Use it to treat dandruff, lice, acne, or herpes.

These are just some of the most common essential oils used by people all over the world. When you buy them, be sure to follow any specific instructions for use. Remember that they are very powerful and heavily concentrated, so a little goes a long way. If you're working with oil you've never used before, it's best to start with a small quantity and slowly add to it if you feel you need more.

Chapter 4: Essential Oil Recipes for Pain Relief

Pain comes in many different forms, from arthritis to migraines to muscle pain. People deal with pain throughout their lives, but you do not have to put up with it. Eliminate pain from your life with these simple essential oil recipes.

Quick Relief Blend for Arthritis

No one should have to deal with joint pain, and you don't have to just deal with your arthritis. This simple blend is easy to make and provides quick relief.

Ingredients:

5 drops Peppermint Oil

4 drops Chamomile Oil

4 drops Eucalyptus Oil

30 ml Carrier Oil (Suggested Sweet Almond Oil)

Directions:

1. Mix together and rub into joints as needed. You'll need to create this mixture each time.

Migraine Remedy

Migraines in different forms plague many people, and all you need for this migraine relief blend is a roller bottle. You should notice relief in just fifteen minutes.

Ingredients:

5 drops Peppermint Oil

5 drops Lavender Oil

Carrier Oil (Suggested Sunflower Oil)

5 drops Rosemary Oil

Directions:

1. Mix all your essential oils together in a roller vial.

2. Next, add your carrier oil until it is full. Shake well.

3. Take a few drops on your fingers and gently massage your forehead, temples, and back of your neck. Keep away from the eyes. Always shake well before using.

Muscle Relaxer

This muscle rub is easy to make and even easier to put on once it's been in a roller bottle. It has a cool, soothing effect, so you'll feel better in as little as ten minutes.

Ingredients:

5 drops Peppermint Oil

3 drops Clove Oil

5 drops Wintergreen Oil

3 drops Black Pepper Oil

Carrier Oil (Suggested Vitamin E)

Directions:

1. Mix all your essential oils in the roller bottle, and then top off with carrier oil.

2. Shake well each time before using. Gently rub the blend into sore areas.

Basic Pain Relief Salve

This is an all-around pain relief salve. It does take about thirty minutes to make, but you'll find you can use it many times. It even keeps up to six to eight months.

Ingredients:

40 drops Eucalyptus Oil

10 drops Rosemary Oil

20 drops Clove Oil

40 drops Peppermint Oil

¼ cup Coconut Oil

¾ cup Sunflower Oil

1 teaspoon Vitamin E Oil

4 tablespoons Beeswax granules

¼ teaspoon Cayenne Pepper

Directions:

1. Use a double boiler, and combine the sunflower oil with the coconut oil. Then add the beeswax over medium heat. Make sure to stir gently until melted.

2. Add your cayenne pepper and stir. Let it cool for five minutes.

3. Add your essential oils and vitamin E oil. Make sure you mix slowly and gently.

4. Pour the mixture into a glass container. Let it cool until the liquid turns into a solid.

5. Store at room temperature.

6. When you want to use it, scoop a small amount, and massage into the painful area.

Chapter 5: Recipes for Cold and Flu

These recipes are great for cold and flu season. You can use them anytime you're feeling down, and most of them can be used right in the diffuser, leaving you with little to no hassle.

Decongestion Blend

One of the worst things about a cold or flu is painful congestion, but as long as you have a diffuser, this blend should help.

Ingredients:

3 drops Peppermint Oil

2 drops Eucalyptus Oil

2 drops Tea Tree Oil

2 drops Lemon Oil

Directions:

1. Put the oils into your diffuser, and use as you normally would.

Sore Throat Soother

Raw honey is extremely important with this recipe. Without it you'll just find irritating sugar in your "honey," which can worsen your sore throat. Local honey is usually best, but you can get organic or raw honey straight from the store.

Ingredients:

1 tablespoon Raw Honey

2 drops Peppermint Oil

1 drop Lemon Oil

Directions:

1. Mix the oils into the honey, and eat as needed.

2. Make sure that all essential oils are food grade before trying this recipe.

Vapor Rub

Remember that vapor rubs will help with congestion and breathing when you have a cold or flu, but not every vapor rub is great for everyone. You'll need to alter the recipe as suggested if you want to use it for children.

Ingredients:

5 tablespoons Coconut Oil

2 tablespoons Cocoa Butter

1½ tablespoons Beeswax Pellets

30 drops Eucalyptus Oil (Eucalyptus Radiata Oil for children)

12 drops Lavender Oil

12 drops Rosemary Oil

12 drops Peppermint Oil

6 drops Tea Tree Oil

Directions:

1. Put a saucepan over low heat, melting your cocoa butter and coconut oil.

2. Add your beeswax once melted, and wait until the beeswax has melted.

3. Take it off the heat, letting it cool. If you don't let it cool, your oils can be damaged.

4. Add your essential oils, combining gently.

5. Pour into a 4-oz. glass container. Once solidified, store at room temperature.

6. Apply to the upper chest as needed.

Homemade Cough Drops

If you're looking for a natural alternative to store-bought cough drops, look no further. Peppermint and spearmint are considered extremely soothing, but you can add other essential oils for flavor. Just make sure you're using food-grade essential oils.

Ingredients:

1 cup Sugar

1 tablespoon Honey

¼ cup Cold Water

Powdered Sugar

10–20 drops Peppermint Oil

10–20 drops Spearmint Oil

Directions:

1. Put the honey, sugar, and water into a bowl, heating over medium heat.

2. Once the temperature reaches 208°F, mix in your essential oils.

3. Once the temperature reaches 300°F, take it off the heat, letting it sit until boiling ceases.

4. Once all the bubbles are gone, put a layer of powdered sugar on a cookie sheet.

5. Take a small spoon and make indents in your sugar, spooning the hot mixture onto the cookie sheet.

6. Let it cool, and then dust off excess sugar.

7. Take when needed.

Stuffy Nose Remedy

Even after your cold or flu has passed, you may still have a stuffy nose. With a diffuser and this essential oil blend, you can get rid of that stuffy nose for good.

Ingredients:

3 drops Peppermint Oil

1 drop Lavender Oil

1 drop Eucalyptus Oil

1 drop Wild Orange Oil

Directions:

1. Put the oils into a diffuser to relieve a stuffy nose.

Chapter 6: Essential Oil Recipes for Acne

Acne isn't something that most people want to talk about, but it is a condition that affects most teens. You do not need to suffer with acne when you can use essential oils to lessen the condition and even get rid of it completely. Remember that different recipes work best for different people. If you have bad luck with one, try another.

Easy Acne Recipe

If you suffer from acne, you don't want to have a ridiculous amount of upkeep. It's best to start with this easy acne recipe to see if it works for you.

Ingredients:

6 drops Frankincense Oil

4 drops Lavender Oil

2 drops Tea Tree Oil

30 ml of Jojoba Oil

Directions:

1. Mix your essential oils with the jojoba oil. Apply to areas that are acne prone right before bed every night.

Blackheads Begone

Many people consider blackheads to be as bad as normal pimples, but there's no reason to fear. This simple baking soda and lemon oil recipe will take care of them in one treatment.

Ingredients:

1 teaspoon Baking Soda

1 teaspoon Water

2–3 drops Lemon Oil

Directions:

1. Mix together until a paste is formed, and apply to the area.

2. Leave it on for twenty to twenty-five minutes before washing off gently.

3. Pat your skin dry.

Pimple Pop Roller

If you don't want to make an acne-fighting recipe every time you need it, just get a roller bottle for this wonderful acne recipe.

Ingredients:

15 drops Tea Tree Oil

15 drops Lavender Oil

15 drops Frankincense Oil

Carrier Oil (Suggested Sweet Almond Oil)

Directions:

1. Combine in a roller bottle, topping the mixture with a carrier oil. A 10-ml roller bottle is suggested.

2. Apply to affected areas or areas of concern before bed each night.

Acne Treatment Cream

Some people are hesitant to put more oil on their acne-prone skin, but this acne-fighting cream will help just as well.

Ingredients:

¼ cup Coconut Oil

10 drops Tea Tree Oil

10 drops Lemon Oil

10 drops Lavender Oil

Directions:

1. Melt your coconut oil before using, and then add the essential oils.

2. Make sure that you don't use a metal spoon. The metal will react with these oils and weaken the strength of your mixture.

3. Put into the refrigerator until firm.

4. Dab on affected areas in both the morning and evening after you clean and dry your face.

Herbal Face Scrub for Acne

Ingredients:

250 ml Oatmeal, finely ground

125 ml Carrier Oil (Suggested Sweet Almond Oil)

1 tablespoon Dry Herbs (Lemongrass, Witch Hazel, Lavender Flowers, or Rose Flower Petals), finely ground

1 teaspoon Spices (Cinnamon Powder or Turmeric Powder)

30 drops Tea Tree Oil

30 drops Lemon Oil

20 drops Lavender Oil

Directions:

1. Mix the ingredients in a widemouthed container with a tight lid.

2. Rub the blend onto your face, but keep away from the eyes. After some time, rinse off with lukewarm water.

Tip: Never scrub your face if you have any swollen acne lacerations.

Chapter 7: Essential Oils for Your Skin

Skincare is a popular reason to use essential oils. People have successfully treated chronic skin conditions, healed wounds, and improved the look and feel of their skin with essential oils. You'll also find body scrubs and moisturizers in this chapter to suit your skin care and beauty needs.

Scar Salve

No one wants to deal with unsightly scars, but you can seldom get rid of scars completely. With this scar salve, however, you can drastically reduce how noticeable the scars are over time.

Ingredients:

20 drops Frankincense Oil

20 drops Helichrysum Oil

20 drops Lavender Oil

1 oz. Beeswax

2 oz. Shea Butter

3 oz. Coconut Oil

Directions:

1. Melt your coconut and Shea butter over medium heat.

2. Add the beeswax, and stir gently until the wax is melted completely. Let it cool for five minutes.

3. Stir in the essential oils.

4. Store in an airtight container. Close your container once the mixture is cool. A 5-oz. container is suggested, as this recipe makes five ounces.

5. Apply two to three times each day.

Whipped Eczema Cream

Eczema is a painful skin condition that spreads if it isn't taken care of properly. Luckily, this eczema cream is both potent and soothing, making it easy to use.

Ingredients:

¼ cup Shea Butter

¼ cup Coconut Oil

15 drops Lavender Oil

5–6 drops Tea Tree Oil

Directions:

1. Using a double boiler, melt your Shea butter as well as your coconut oil.

2. Remove from the heat and let cool for up to five minutes.

3. Gently add all your oils before scooping the mixture into a bowl.

4. Beat on high until whipped, and spoon into a glass jar.

5. Rub onto affected areas twice a day.

Moisturizing your skin is important for its health. If you have properly moisturized skin, it'll appear softer and even brighter.

Ingredients:

1¾ cup Unrefined Shea Butter

½ cup Extra Virgin Coconut Oil

¼ cup Grapeseed Oil

20 drops Sweet Orange Oil

15 drops Lemon Oil

Directions:

1. Add your coconut oil and unrefined Shea butter to a double boiler. You'll need to melt it slowly, stirring constantly so that there are no lumps.

2. Let cool slightly before adding your grapeseed oil and essential oils.

3. Let cool until solid again, and then whip on high.

4. Put into a glass jar, and apply to skin to moisturize it and relax tense muscles.

Wrinkle Cream

You don't have to be old to get wrinkles. Actually, different people will get wrinkles at different times, but no matter your age, you can benefit from this wrinkle-reduction cream.

Ingredients:

¼ cup Shea Butter

¼ cup Organic Coconut Oil

7–10 drops Lavender Oil

10–12 drops Frankincense Oil

Directions:

1. Melt your coconut oil and Shea butter. It's best to use a double boiler, and then let it cool.

2. Make sure you gently add your essential oils, mixing completely.

3. Let the mixture cool to room temperature, and apply each night before bed to reduce wrinkles. It should be applied after cleaning your face and patting it dry.

Stretch Mark Reducing Blend

Stretch marks can make people feel uncomfortable with their bodies, but you can reduce the visibility of stretch marks with this recipe.

Ingredients:

5 drops Frankincense Oil

5 drops Myrrh Oil

5 drops Grapefruit Oil

¼ cup Coconut Oil

Directions:

1. Melt your coconut oil before mixing in your essential oils.

2. Let it cool, and apply to stretch marks up to three times daily.

Natural Toner

Everyone can benefit from a toner to eliminate excess toxins and oils, but not everyone has the money to spend for this treatment. This essential oil toner, however, is cheap and easy to make.

Ingredients:

8 oz. Water

2 drops Lavender Oil

2 drops Geranium Oil

2 drops Frankincense Oil

Directions:

1. Mix together and put into a bottle.

2. Shake well before using, and dip a cotton ball into it to apply gently to your skin. Only apply after washing and patting your face dry.

Oil Blend for Age Spots

No matter your age, you'll find that you have some sort of blemish. These blemishes can turn into age spots as you get older, and no one wants to deal with that. By just using this one essential oil correctly, you can reduce your age spots in no time at all.

Ingredients:

6 drops Frankincense Oil

½ teaspoon Vitamin E Oil

Directions:

1. Mix and apply directly to your skin.

Sweet Sugar Scrub

This sugar scrub is meant to exfoliate skin, making it softer and brighter. You should not allow dead skin cells to pile up and make your skin look bad and feel even worse.

Ingredients:

2 cups White Sugar

½ cup Coconut Oil, melted

7–10 drops Orange Oil

3–5 drops Vanilla Extract

Directions:

1. Combine the sugar and coconut oil in a bowl.

2. Add the orange oil and vanilla extract. Stir to mix well.

3. Store the mixture in a widemouthed container with a tight lid.

4. Scrub the blend over the skin to exfoliate and cleanse, keeping away from the eyes.

5. Rinse away with warm water and pat dry.

Bath Bomb for Skin Care

Ingredients:

2 cups Baking Soda

1 cup Sea Salt

1 cup Citric Acid

1 cup Corn Starch

1 tablespoon Jojoba Oil

30 drops Tea Tree Oil

30 drops Lemon Oil

20 drops Lavender Oil

60 ml Witch Hazel in a Spray Bottle

Directions:

1. Mix all the ingredients except the witch hazel in a container.

2. While mixing, moisten the mixture with the witch hazel spray.

3. Pack the mixture into ice cube molds, and let them dry overnight.

4. Take the bath bombs out of the molds, and air-dry for two more days before using them in your bath.

Chapter 8: Essential Oils for Lip Care

Most people don't think about their lips when they think about essential oils. Even when trying homemade health and beauty remedies, lips are often forgotten. With these essential oil recipes, however, you'll find that your lips will look plumper, softer, and healthier.

Homemade Lip Balm

Lip balm is essential to lip health, especially if you want supple and soft lips, which will make it easier to apply makeup later. You can trade out the essential oil for lemon or peppermint for a more soothing mixture.

Ingredients:

5 tablespoons Coconut Oil

3 tablespoons Beeswax

12 drops Orange Oil

Directions:

1. Using a double boiler, melt your beeswax and coconut oil.

2. While it's hot, add the orange oil.

3. Pour into lip balm tubes. Let the tubes cool at room temperature before capping them.

Peppermint Lip Scrub

Peppermint is invigorating, and in this lip scrub, it'll help make sure that you get rid of any dead skin cells so that your lips stay soft and kissable.

Ingredients:

1 teaspoon Coconut Oil

1 teaspoon Raw Honey

3 drops Peppermint Oil

1½ teaspoons White Sugar

Directions:

1. Mix all your ingredients together in a bowl.

2. Put into a container.

3. When you want to use it, gently scrub over lips and rinse with warm water to exfoliate.

DIY Plumper

There's no reason to spend a large amount of money on chemical-laced plumping serums. You can make your own lips plumper right at home with essential oils by using this natural recipe.

Ingredients:

1 Vitamin E Capsule

6 drops Cinnamon Oil

2 drops Olive Oil

1 teaspoon Beeswax

Directions:

1. Melt your beeswax in your double boiler. You'll need to stir occasionally and then add your olive oil.

2. Break open the vitamin E oil capsule and mix it in gently.

3. Once it starts to cool down, add your cinnamon oil, and stir.

4. Pour into a jar, and let it cool before sealing.

5. Gently apply over lips with fingertips. Rinse with warm water.

Healing Lip Balm

This healing lip balm is great for chapped or even cracked lips. It'll keep your lips soft while healing them as well.

Ingredients:

2 tablespoons Calendula Petals, dried

2 tablespoons Marshmallow Root

3 tablespoons Beeswax

¼ cup Extra Virgin Coconut Oil

5 drops Peppermint Oil

5 drops Lavender Oil

Directions:

1. Melt your coconut oil, and add your herbs.

2. Let it all sit together over low heat for about four to five minutes before placing into a warm oven.

3. Let it steep for three to four hours before straining out the herbs.

4. Put the strained oil back over low heat, adding your wax to melt.

5. Add the essential oils, and make sure you mix completely.

6. Pour into containers to use as needed.

Cold Sore Treatment

Cold sores are painful when they occur, but they often occur right on your lips or outside of them. You can quickly get rid of a cold sore with this helpful essential oil remedy.

Ingredients:

3 drops Lemon Balm Oil

2 drops Tea Tree Oil

3 drops Lavender Oil

3 drops Eucalyptus Oil

3 drops Roman Chamomile Oil

3 drops Bergamot Oil

4 drops Geranium Oil

1 oz. Sweet Almond Oil

Directions:

1. Put the essential oils into a roller bottle and mix.

2. Add one to two drops of the blend on a Q-tip and dab on sore spots.

Chapter 9: Essential Oil Recipes for Hair Care

From helping an itchy scalp, getting rid of dandruff, and renewing hair growth to ridding yourself of lice naturally, essential oils can help. With these wonderful recipes, you can take care of your hair in no time.

Itchy Scalp Remedy

An itchy scalp can strike at any time, but what most people don't realize is that an itchy scalp means an unhealthy scalp. Use this essential oil mixture to heal your scalp.

Ingredients:

15 drops Lavender Oil

15 drops Lemon Oil

10 drops Tea Tree Oil

1½ cups Water

1/2 cup Witch Hazel

Directions:

1. Mix everything together in a spray bottle, and mist your hair after washing or before brushing. You can do this two to three times daily.

Anti-Dandruff Shampoo

Dandruff can be caused by a variety of things, but no matter the cause, this anti-dandruff recipe can help. With lavender essential oil, you'll even get a soothing effect to help after a long, stressful day.

Ingredients:

5 drops Tea Tree Oil

2 drops Lavender Oil

1 drop Rosemary Oil

2 drops Copaiba Oil

Directions:

1. Add the essential oils to your shampoo treatment for that day (not the bottle).

2. Apply directly to your scalp, and let it sit for one to two minutes before washing.

Dry Scalp Cure

Dry scalp can cause an itchy scalp, but it can also just be a pain all on its own. This recipe is easy to make and easy to use. You can even mix it into your conditioner.

Ingredients:

6 drops Cedarwood Oil

2 drops Patchouli Oil

2 drops Geranium Oil

1 teaspoon Coconut Oil

Directions:

1. Mix everything together, and massage gently into your dry scalp.

2. Cover with a towel for a minimum of fifteen minutes, and then shampoo and thoroughly rinse your hair twice.

Deep Hair Conditioner

You don't need to pay salon prices to get a deep conditioning treatment that works without the chemicals. You'll find that this all-natural, essential oil–infused recipe does wonders for the health and shine of your hair.

Ingredients:

15 drops Rosewood Oil

9 drops Sandalwood Oil

9 drops Lavender Oil

½ cup Olive Oil

Directions:

1. Mix everything together in a bag, and warm up gently in warm water by dunking the bag into it.

2. Apply it to your hair, wrapping your hair for twenty to twenty-five minutes.

3. Shampoo and wash your hair as usual.

Hair Moisturizer

Ingredients:

1 oz. Jojoba Oil (if you have black hair, use Camellia Oil)

12 drops Cedarwood Oil

12 drops Lavender Oil

8 drops Rosemary Oil

Directions:

1. Combine all the ingredients in a PET plastic bottle.

2. After mixing them well, massage about a teaspoonful of the combination into your hair and scalp.

3. Use a shower cap and wrap it all using a warm moistened towel. Wait for a minimum of fifteen minutes, and then shampoo and thoroughly rinse your hair twice.

4. Dry it and then style it as you normally do. This can be done weekly or monthly.

Beard Oil Recipe

If you have a beard or just want to give the gift of all-natural beard oil, this recipe is great for you. Beard hair can be hard to tame, but this recipe will make it smoother and more manageable.

Ingredients:

½ oz. Argon Oil

¼ oz. Sweet Almond Oil

¼ oz. Jojoba Oil

7 drops Lavender Oil

5 drops Rosemary Oil

3 drops Cedarwood Oil

Directions:

1. Mix together and put into a glass bottle that has a dropper.

2. Drop three to five drops into your hand, and work through your beard. If you have a longer beard, you may need more drops, but add a small amount at a time so that you do not oversaturate the hair.

DIY Lice Treatment

Unfortunately, lice affect many people no matter how hard they try to avoid them, but you don't need to rely on chemical-laced shampoos if you use this essential oil treatment.

Ingredients:

1 cup Olive Oil

20 drops Tea Tree Oil

20 drops Lavender Oil

Directions:

1. Mix together and apply to your hair.

2. Leave the mixture on for an hour before combing your hair.

3. Shampoo twice to rinse the mixture completely.

Chapter 10: Essential Oil Recipes for Reducing Anxiety, Insomnia, and Fatigue

Essential oils have many emotional benefits when used in the right blends. This chapter is dedicated to helping you relieve anxiety, insomnia, fatigue, and so much more. Essential oils can affect your mood, helping to improve your life.

Soothing Blend for Anxiety

There's no shame in having anxiety, but you shouldn't sit back and do nothing. To get rid of anxiety naturally, you'll find that this simple blend helps immensely.

Ingredients:

10 drops Lavender Oil

4 drops Rosemary Oil

Directions:

1. Diffuse the oils in a diffuser as you would normally to reduce stress.

Relaxing Blend for Stress Relief

Ingredients:

30 drops Cedarwood Oil

30 drops Ylang Ylang Oil

25 drops Lavender Oil

20 drops Patchouli Oil

20 drops Bergamot Oil

Jojoba Oil (optional)

Directions:

1. Mix all the essential oils in a dark glass vial. Dilute the mixture with the jojoba oil if desired.

2. Take a few drops and rub them between your palms and deeply inhale the scent for an immediate calming effect when you are in anxious or stressful situations.

3. You can add a few drops to warm bathwater for a peaceful and tranquilizing bath.

Lavender Remedy for Insomnia

Insomnia often hits at the worst possible time. You can't do much about it besides trying to relax, but you only need one essential oil to help you relax enough to kick insomnia out of your life.

Ingredients:

Lavender Oil

Directions:

1. Just put a few drops of lavender oil on your pillow and you'll rest a little easier.

2. Reapply once a week.

Relaxing is a great way to improve your mood because tension will make for a bad day and even a severe headache. You'll notice the effects of this remedy in as little as five minutes.

Ingredients:

½ teaspoon Sweet Almond Oil

2–4 drops Chamomile Oil

4 drops Lavender Oil

3 drops Peppermint Oil

Directions:

1. Mix together and apply directly to your temples.

Calm a Child

Children can be hard to calm down, and they have bad days just like adults. This essential oil blend is great to keep on hand, and you can use it in advance to keep your children calm and happy.

Ingredients:

25 drops Chamomile Oil

25 drops Lavender Oil

½ cup Water

Directions:

1. Put into a spritzer bottle, and spray on stuffed animals or bedding to help calm upset children.

Fatigue takes a toll on mental health, making it difficult to get through the day when you're tired. This essential oil blend will help relax you but wake you up at the same time.

Ingredients:

10 drops Peppermint Oil

4–5 drops Lemongrass Oil

Directions:

1. Add to a diffuser, and inhale to relieve fatigue.

Chapter 11: Essential Oil Recipes for Allergies, Sunburn, and Blisters

There is so much more that you can do with essential oils. You can use them to boost your immune system, help relieve allergies, and heal blisters.

Allergy Relief

Allergies can affect you at the worst times and even cause problems throughout the year for certain individuals. Not everyone wants to take allergy medicine or even has it on hand, but certain essential oils can relieve the worst of the symptoms.

Ingredients:

¼ teaspoon Sweet Almond Oil

2 drops Lavender Oil

3 drops Frankincense Oil

Directions:

1. Mix together and rub on your palms before inhaling deeply. This should help relieve allergy symptoms, such as itchy eyes and throat irritation.

Poison Ivy Treatment

Poison ivy is a difficult ailment to deal with, but you'll find relief quickly and effectively with this blend, which is also effective for treating poison oak.

48

Ingredients:

3 drops Peppermint Oil

½ teaspoon Coconut Oil

Directions:

1. Melt the coconut oil, and mix in the essential oil.

2. Using a cotton ball, apply the blend to the affected area three times a day.

Essential Oil Remedy for Sunburn

Sunburn can happen at any time of the year, and severity will always vary. This essential oil blend will help provide quick, soothing relief.

Ingredients:

1 tablespoon Coconut Oil

7 drops Lavender Oil

7 drops Chamomile Oil

Directions:

1. Melt your coconut oil, and mix in your essential oils.

2. When cooled down, apply to your sunburn with a cotton ball. This should help reduce the swelling and pain.

Immune Booster

Everyone could use a boost to their immune system, and this essential oil treatment can be helpful.

Ingredients:

2 drops Oregano Oil

6 drops Sweet Almond Oil

Directions:

1. Mix together and rub on the bottom of your feet.

2. Apply at least once each day.

Healing Blend for Blisters

Blisters can develop from burns and even physical duress. It doesn't matter what type of blister you have because this essential oil blend can help heal and soothe it. You can even make a large amount and keep it on hand if you have a roller bottle.

Ingredients:

2 drops Tea Tree Oil

2 drops Vitamin E Oil

Directions:

1. Mix together and apply to the blisters four to five times daily.

Chapter 12: Essential Oil Baths

You can also just use essential oils in a bath and soak your problems away. You'll need to make sure you use the right blends for your problems. These baths can help you chase away headaches, congestion, and even just everyday anxiety.

Sinus Decongestion Blend

Sinus congestion can be eliminated with an essential oil bath, but make sure you don't splash this bath into your eyes.

Ingredients:

1 cup Epsom Salt

½ cup Baking Soda

10 drops Eucalyptus Oil

5 drops Peppermint Oil

Directions:

1. Mix all the ingredients in a container before placing in hot bathwater.

2. Relax in the bath for twenty minutes. You can use the mixture all at once or just half at a time.

Stress Relieving Bath

You should use this mixture once a week, and make sure that you soak for at least twenty minutes. It'll help lower your stress-related hormones, balance your pH level, and even pull out toxins.

Ingredients:

½ cup Epsom Salt

10 drops Lavender Oil

½ cup Baking Soda

4 drops Rose Oil

Directions:

1. Mix the ingredients together, and put into warm bathwater.

2. Soak for twenty minutes, and then continue your bath like normal.

Sleepy Time Bath

Maybe it hasn't gotten as far as insomnia, but you'll find that poor sleep creates a bad mood. Luckily, this bath is designed to help you to relax enough to get a good night's rest right afterward.

Ingredients:

10 drops Lavender Oil

7 drops Roman Chamomile Oil

¼ cup Sea Salt

1 tablespoon Jojoba Oil

Directions:

1. Mix everything together, and then add to a warm bath. Soak for about twenty minutes.

Relaxing Bath for Anxiety

Anxiety strikes at any time, and it can build up if you don't do anything about it. With this bath, you can melt anxiety away, clearing your mind and relaxing your muscles.

Ingredients:

10 drops Frankincense Oil

5 drops Bergamot Oil

1 cup Full Fat Milk

5 drops Lavender Oil

Directions:

1. Mix it all together before combining with your hot bathwater, soaking for about an hour.

Stress Relief Bath

Stress is just as bad as anxiety and can even lead to depression. It's important to deal with stress and let it go, which is what this essential oil bath helps you to do.

Ingredients:

10 drops Rose Oil

10 drops Frankincense Oil

2 tablespoons Coconut Oil

¼ cup Sea Salt

Directions:

1. Mix it all together before applying to your warm bathwater. Soak for about thirty minutes.

Soothing Bath for Muscle Tension

Muscle tension doesn't always need a cream. You'll find that this bath can help just as much, and it's a lot easier to use when you don't feel like doing anything but soaking your troubles away.

Ingredients:

10 drops Lavender Oil

5 drops Peppermint Oil

5 drops Citrus Oil

3 drops Clove Oil

1 tablespoon Jojoba Oil

Directions:

1. Mix all the ingredients together before adding to your bathwater, and then soak for at least thirty minutes.

Headache Relief Bath

Headaches come in many forms, but this essential oil bath is just meant to target the most basic kind. It isn't for migraines, but it'll help with any headaches that might turn into one if not treated.

Ingredients:

1 tablespoon Sesame Seed Oil

5 drops Eucalyptus Oil

10 drops Peppermint Oil

Directions:

1. Mix all the ingredients together before adding to warm bathwater.

2. Soak for about thirty to forty minutes. Be careful not to splash it in your eyes, as it can cause irritation. If you do, just rinse immediately.

Aromatherapy Bath for Migraines

This bath recipe is for a migraine or headache that is due to hormonal problems or lack of sleep. When used for the proper migraine, it should help immensely.

Ingredients:

5 drops Sandalwood Oil

2 tablespoons Baking Soda

1 tablespoon Jojoba Oil

10 drops Chamomile Oil

10 drops Peppermint Oil

Directions:

1. Mix all ingredients together, and then put into warm bathwater. Soak for about thirty minutes or more.

Clarity Bath

This bath is meant to help you focus your mind and find clarity on anything you're struggling with. This wonderful essential oil blend benefits you mentally.

Ingredients:

5 drops Cedarwood Oil

5 drops Sandalwood Oil

2 tablespoons Jojoba Oil

10 drops Vetiver Oil

Directions:

1. Combine everything before mixing it into the warm bathwater, soaking for at least thirty minutes.

Allergy Relief Bath

With this wonderful bath, you'll find that your allergies wouldn't bother you. It's a great way to start or end your day to get the relief you need during the worst days of any allergy season.

Ingredients:

¼ cup Epsom Salt

1 tablespoon Sesame Seed Oil

5 drops Basil Oil

10 drops Lavender Oil

Directions:

1. Combine all ingredients before adding to the warm bathwater, soaking for at least twenty minutes.

Conclusion

As you have seen, including essential oils in your daily life is easy. From helping you get fuller, shinier hair to helping you with that much needed allergy relief during allergy season, essential oils are there for you. It is important for you to learn all the properties of essential oils before using them. With essential oils, you will always have all-natural remedies for a wide range of ailments and conditions at your fingertips, and you will be able to avoid toxic chemicals that are often included in commercial products.

Keep in mind that essential oils last from one to three years, and they need to be stored in dark glass bottles. Also, when you mix essential oils with a carrier oil, they will usually not last more than three months.

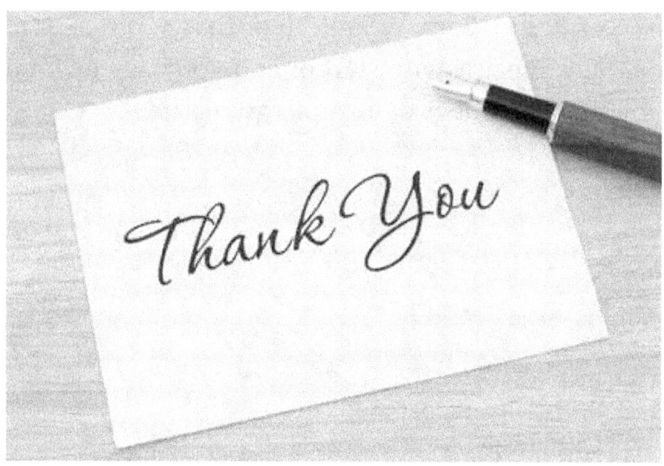

Finally, I want to thank you for reading my book. If you enjoyed the book, please share your thoughts and post a review on the book retailer's website. It would be greatly appreciated!

Best wishes,

Savannah Gibbs

www.ingramcontent.com/pod-product-compliance
Lightning Source LLC
Chambersburg PA
CBHW061714130726
47996CB00006B/2311